REVEALING THE KEYS TO EPILEPSY AND SEIZURE RECOVERY

A Comprehensive Guide to Reclaiming Control and Embracing a Life Beyond Seizures

David Benson

Table of contents

Introduction

Understanding Epilepsy

Understanding epilepsy is a crucial step in navigating the complexities of this neurological disorder. Epilepsy, often characterized by recurrent seizures, is not a singular condition but a spectrum of disorders affecting the brain's electrical activity. To truly comprehend epilepsy, one must delve into its diverse manifestations, causes, and the impact it has on individuals' lives.

At its core, epilepsy is defined by the occurrence of seizures—sudden, uncontrolled electrical disturbances in the brain. These seizures can manifest in various ways, from brief lapses of consciousness to convulsions affecting the entire body. It is important to recognize that epilepsy is not a mental illness, nor is it a sign of intellectual impairment. Instead, it is a neurological condition stemming from abnormal brain activity.

Seizures occur due to disruptions in the intricate balance of electrical signals between nerve cells in the brain. This can be caused by a multitude of factors, including genetic predispositions, brain injuries, infections, or structural abnormalities in the brain. Understanding the root causes of epilepsy is essential for accurate diagnosis and effective management.

The diagnosis of epilepsy is often a complex process that involves thorough medical history reviews, neurological examinations, and diagnostic tests such as EEGs (electroencephalograms) to monitor brain activity. It is crucial to distinguish between isolated seizures and epilepsy, as not everyone who experiences a seizure has the disorder. Recurrent, unprovoked seizures are a key indicator of epilepsy.

Living with epilepsy goes beyond the physical manifestation of seizures; it profoundly influences various aspects of daily life. Individuals with epilepsy may face challenges in education, employment, and social interactions due to the unpredictable nature of seizures. Understanding the impact of epilepsy on a person's life is fundamental to offering support and fostering a more inclusive society.

Moreover, epilepsy is not a one-size-fits-all condition. The diversity in seizure types and triggers underscores the need for personalized treatment plans. Antiepileptic medications are commonly prescribed to control seizures, but their efficacy varies from person to person. Some may require a combination of medications, while others might explore alternative therapies such as dietary changes or neurostimulation devices.

In addition to medical interventions, lifestyle modifications play a pivotal role in managing epilepsy. Nutrition, sleep patterns, and stress levels can significantly influence seizure frequency. For many individuals, identifying and addressing these factors can be as crucial as medication in achieving seizure control.

Understanding epilepsy extends beyond the individual diagnosed; it encompasses their support network. Family, friends, and colleagues can contribute significantly to an individual's well-being by being informed and empathetic. Education and awareness campaigns play a vital role in dispelling misconceptions and reducing the stigma associated with epilepsy, fostering a more supportive environment for those affected.

Embracing technology and innovation is another aspect of understanding epilepsy in contemporary times. Wearable devices and mobile applications can aid in tracking seizures, medication adherence, and overall health, empowering individuals to actively participate in their care and providing valuable data for healthcare professionals.

Understanding epilepsy is a multifaceted journey that involves grasping the neurological intricacies, acknowledging the impact on daily life, and fostering a supportive environment. By unraveling the complexities of epilepsy, society can move towards a more inclusive and compassionate approach, ensuring that individuals affected by this condition receive the understanding and support they deserve.

The Road to Recovery

Embarking on the road to recovery from epilepsy is a journey filled with challenges, victories, and profound self-discovery. This chapter delves into the intricacies of this path, guiding individuals through the various stages and highlighting the essential components that contribute to a successful recovery.

Understanding the Landscape:

The journey begins with a deep understanding of epilepsy—the neurological condition characterized by recurrent seizures. By unraveling the scientific aspects of seizures and their impact on daily life, individuals gain insight into the nature of their condition. This knowledge serves as the foundation for informed decision-making and empowers individuals to take an active role in their recovery.

Acceptance and Resilience:

One of the initial milestones on the road to recovery is acceptance. Acceptance does not imply surrendering to the condition but rather acknowledging it as a part of one's life. Embracing resilience is equally crucial—recognizing that setbacks may occur but can be overcome with determination and perseverance. This mental shift lays the groundwork for a positive and proactive approach to managing epilepsy.

Navigating the Diagnostic Process:
The journey continues with a thorough exploration of the diagnostic process. Navigating through medical tests, consultations, and obtaining a clear diagnosis is a critical step. Understanding the nuances of diagnostic tools and engaging in open communication with healthcare professionals ensures that individuals are equipped with the knowledge needed to make informed decisions about their treatment.

Medications and Beyond:
Treatment options, particularly medications, play a pivotal role in seizure management. This section provides insights into various antiepileptic drugs, their mechanisms, and potential side effects. It also explores alternative therapies, recognizing that a holistic approach to recovery may include complementary practices such as acupuncture, dietary changes, or herbal supplements.

Lifestyle Modifications for Seizure Control:

The road to recovery involves a commitment to lifestyle changes that contribute to seizure control. Exploring the impact of nutrition, regular exercise, and stress management techniques empowers individuals to proactively manage triggers and enhance overall well-being. This section acts as a practical guide, offering tips and strategies to incorporate these changes into daily life.

Building a Support System:

No journey is undertaken alone, and the road to epilepsy recovery is no exception. Building a robust support system is a key component. This chapter explores the roles of family, friends, and healthcare providers in creating a network that fosters understanding, encouragement, and assistance. It also emphasizes the benefits of connecting with epilepsy support groups, where individuals can share experiences and gain valuable insights.

Empowering the Mind:

Recovery extends beyond the physical aspects of epilepsy; it involves empowering the mind. Techniques such as mindfulness, meditation, and cognitive behavioral strategies are powerful tools in managing stress, anxiety, and emotional challenges. This section guides individuals in cultivating a positive mindset, setting realistic goals, and harnessing the mind's resilience.

Overcoming Challenges:
Challenges are inevitable on the road to recovery, and this chapter addresses them head-on. From navigating societal stigma to coping with emotional struggles and addressing employment and social hurdles, individuals are equipped with strategies to overcome obstacles and emerge stronger on the other side.

Seizure Safety and First Aid:
Safety is a paramount concern for those living with epilepsy. This section provides practical advice on creating a safe environment and offers essential first aid tips for seizures. Empowering individuals and their support networks with this knowledge enhances confidence and preparedness in handling potential challenges.

Flourishing Beyond Epilepsy:
The final leg of the journey is marked by a celebration of achievements and a look toward the

future. Embracing a positive mindset, pursuing personal dreams, and drawing inspiration from the triumphs of others propel individuals toward a future filled with possibilities.

In conclusion, the road to recovery from epilepsy is a transformative journey that encompasses understanding, acceptance, and proactive management. With the right knowledge, support, and mindset, individuals can navigate this road with resilience, emerging stronger and more empowered on the other side.

The Science Behind Seizures

Unraveling the Neurological Puzzle

Epilepsy, a condition characterized by recurrent seizures, is a complex neurological puzzle that demands understanding at both scientific and personal levels. In this chapter, we embark on a journey to decipher the intricate workings of the brain during seizures, aiming to shed light on the mystery that shrouds epilepsy.

The human brain, a marvel of complexity, consists of billions of neurons communicating through intricate networks. Epileptic seizures result from abnormal electrical discharges in the brain, disrupting this delicate dance of neural signals. To unravel this neurological puzzle, it is crucial to comprehend the basics of brain function and the factors that can trigger seizures.

At its core, epilepsy arises from an imbalance in the delicate interplay of excitatory and inhibitory signals in the brain. Neurons communicate through electrical impulses, and an epileptic brain experiences a surge of abnormal electrical activity.

This can manifest in various forms, from brief lapses in awareness to convulsive movements. Understanding the specific mechanisms that lead to these seizures is essential for cffcctive management and recovery.

The journey begins with an exploration of the brain's regions and their roles in seizure genesis. We delve into the hippocampus, amygdala, and other key structures, unraveling how abnormalities in these areas can contribute to epileptic activity. Mapping the brain's geography provides valuable insights into the diverse manifestations of seizures and helps tailor treatment approaches to individual needs.

As we navigate the complexities of neuronal communication, we encounter neurotransmitters – the messengers that relay signals between neurons. Imbalances in neurotransmitter levels can tip the scales toward hyperexcitability, setting the stage for seizures. Gaining an understanding of these chemical messengers equips individuals and their healthcare teams with the knowledge to explore targeted interventions for seizure control.

Genetics, another piece of the puzzle, plays a significant role in epilepsy. By unraveling the intricate genetic landscape, researchers aim to identify specific genes associated with epilepsy and its various forms. This genetic insight not only enhances diagnostic precision but also opens avenues for personalized treatment strategies tailored to an individual's unique genetic makeup.

Beyond genetics, environmental factors contribute to the complexity of epilepsy. Traumatic brain injuries, infections, and exposure to certain substances can act as triggers, pushing the neurological system toward a seizure threshold. Uncovering these environmental influences helps individuals with epilepsy make informed lifestyle choices to minimize risks and optimize their overall well-being.

In our exploration of the neurological puzzle, we encounter the concept of epileptogenesis – the process by which a normal brain transitions to a hyperexcitable state prone to seizures. Unraveling this process provides a roadmap for intervention at various stages, offering hope for preventing the development or progression of epilepsy in susceptible individuals.

In the latter part of this chapter, we delve into advanced neuroimaging techniques such as magnetic resonance imaging (MRI) and electroencephalography (EEG). These tools allow healthcare professionals to visualize and monitor the brain's activity, aiding in the diagnosis and ongoing management of epilepsy. By understanding the patterns and abnormalities revealed through neuroimaging, individuals gain valuable insights into their condition, fostering a sense of empowerment in their journey toward recovery.

"Unraveling the Neurological Puzzle" serves as a cornerstone in comprehending epilepsy, bridging the gap between the intricacies of brain function and the individual experience of living with seizures. Armed with this knowledge, individuals can actively engage in their treatment plans, foster open communication with healthcare providers, and navigate the path to recovery with newfound understanding and resilience.

Types of Seizures Explained

Seizures, characterized by abnormal electrical activity in the brain, manifest in various forms and intensities. Understanding the different types of seizures is crucial for individuals affected by epilepsy, as it guides both medical professionals and those providing support. This comprehensive exploration aims to shed light on the diverse landscape of seizures.

1. Tonic-Clonic Seizures:

Formerly known as grand mal seizures, these are perhaps the most widely recognized type. Tonic-Clonic seizures involve two distinct phases. The tonic phase involves the sudden stiffening of muscles, causing the person to fall if standing. This is followed by the clonic phase, marked by rhythmic, jerking muscle movements. Tonic-Clonic seizures are often accompanied by altered consciousness, and individuals may experience confusion or fatigue afterward.

2. Absence Seizures:

Formerly referred to as petit mal seizures, absence seizures are characterized by brief lapses in consciousness. The person may appear to be staring into space, exhibiting minimal movement. These episodes are often so subtle that they can be mistaken for daydreaming. Absence seizures are more common in children and typically last for a few seconds.

3. Complex Partial Seizures:
These seizures originate in a specific area of the brain and can cause a range of complex behaviors. Individuals may exhibit repetitive movements, gestures, or even engage in purposeless activities during the seizure. Complex partial seizures often involve altered consciousness and may leave the person confused or disoriented afterward.

4. Simple Partial Seizures:
In contrast to complex partial seizures, simple partial seizures do not result in altered consciousness. They may, however, cause unusual sensations, movements, or emotions. The symptoms experienced depend on the specific region of the brain affected. Simple partial seizures can serve as a warning sign, indicating the potential for more severe seizures.

5. Myoclonic Seizures:

Myoclonic seizures are characterized by sudden, brief jerks or twitches of the arms and legs. These seizures can be isolated events or part of a more extensive seizure disorder. While they may be mistaken for normal muscle twitches, the repetitive and sudden nature distinguishes myoclonic seizures.

6. Atonic Seizures:

Atonic seizures, also known as drop attacks, involve a sudden loss of muscle tone. The individual may collapse or slump, sometimes leading to falls. Atonic seizures are brief and typically last for only a few seconds. Protective measures, such as helmets, may be recommended for those prone to atonic seizures to prevent injuries.

7. Clonic Seizures:

Clonic seizures are characterized by rhythmic, jerking muscle movements. These seizures may affect a specific part of the body or involve the entire body. Clonic seizures often occur during the tonic-clonic phase of a seizure but can also manifest independently.

8. Focal Onset Impaired Awareness Seizures:

Formerly known as complex partial seizures with secondary generalization, these seizures originate in a specific area of the brain and may evolve into tonic-clonic seizures. The impaired awareness during the seizure can lead to unusual behaviors, automatisms, or even purposeful movements.

In understanding these diverse seizure types, it's essential to recognize that epilepsy is a spectrum disorder. Each person's experience is unique, and seizures can manifest differently across individuals. The classification of seizures aids in diagnosis, treatment planning, and the development of appropriate strategies for seizure management.

Individuals with epilepsy, along with their caregivers, benefit from education and awareness about these various seizure types. This knowledge not only promotes a deeper understanding of the condition but also empowers individuals to actively participate in their treatment plans, leading to better seizure control and an improved quality of life.

Diagnosis and Treatment Options

Navigating the Diagnostic Process

Navigating the diagnostic process when facing epilepsy can be a complex and often emotional journey. This phase is crucial for understanding the nature of the condition, determining appropriate treatment, and developing a plan for recovery. In this chapter, we will explore the key aspects of navigating the diagnostic process.

1. Initial Concerns and Seeking Medical Advice:
The journey typically begins with the recognition of unusual symptoms or behaviors that may indicate a seizure. Individuals or their loved ones often notice episodes of unexplained staring, repetitive movements, or loss of consciousness. When such concerns arise, seeking medical advice promptly is essential. Primary care physicians are often the first point of contact, conducting preliminary evaluations and referring patients to specialists if necessary.

2. Neurological Evaluation:

A crucial step in the diagnostic process is a thorough neurological evaluation by a specialist, such as a neurologist or epileptologist. This involves a comprehensive medical history, detailed discussions about the observed symptoms, and a physical examination. The neurologist may also order various diagnostic tests to gather more information about the brain's activity.

3. Diagnostic Tests:

To confirm the presence of epilepsy and identify the specific type of seizures, diagnostic tests are employed. The most common test is an Electroencephalogram (EEG), which records the brain's electrical activity. Other imaging studies, such as Magnetic Resonance Imaging (MRI) and Computed Tomography (CT) scans, may also be conducted to identify any structural abnormalities in the brain.

4. Monitoring and Recording Seizure Activity:

In some cases, long-term monitoring may be necessary to capture the frequency and patterns of seizures. This can be achieved through video EEG monitoring, where patients stay in a specialized unit for an extended period while their brain activity and behavior are continuously recorded. This helps healthcare professionals gain a more in-depth understanding of the seizures and aids in accurate diagnosis.

5. Interpreting Test Results:

Once the diagnostic tests are completed, the neurologist interprets the results and makes a diagnosis. It's important for individuals to actively engage in discussions with their healthcare team, seeking clarification on any aspects they find confusing. Understanding the diagnosis lays the foundation for informed decision-making regarding treatment options.

6. Coping with Emotional Impact:

The diagnostic process is not only a physical journey but an emotional one as well. Receiving an epilepsy diagnosis can be overwhelming, and individuals may experience a range of emotions, including fear, anxiety, and uncertainty about the future. Providing emotional support and resources during this phase is crucial for helping individuals cope with the emotional impact of the diagnosis.

7. Exploring Treatment Options:

Once a diagnosis is confirmed, the next step involves exploring appropriate treatment options. The choice of treatment depends on factors such as the type of seizures, their frequency, and the individual's overall health. Treatment options may include antiepileptic medications, lifestyle modifications, or, in some cases, surgical interventions. Engaging in open and honest discussions with the healthcare team is vital for making informed decisions about the best course of action.

8. Ongoing Monitoring and Adjustments:

Managing epilepsy is often an ongoing process that requires regular monitoring and adjustments to the treatment plan. Periodic check-ups with healthcare providers help assess the effectiveness of the chosen treatment and make any necessary modifications to optimize seizure control while minimizing side effects.

Navigating the diagnostic process in epilepsy is a collaborative effort between individuals, their families, and healthcare professionals. It involves a blend of medical expertise, emotional support, and informed decision-making to lay the groundwork for a comprehensive and effective recovery journey.

Medications and Their Impact

Medications play a crucial role in managing epilepsy, aiming to control seizures and enhance the quality of life for individuals affected by this neurological condition. The impact of epilepsy medications is multifaceted, encompassing not only seizure control but also potential side effects, adherence challenges, and the ongoing quest for optimal treatment.

1. Controlling Seizures:
Epilepsy medications, also known as antiepileptic drugs (AEDs), primarily work by stabilizing electrical activity in the brain to prevent abnormal and excessive firing of neurons that lead to seizures. These drugs target various mechanisms involved in the generation and propagation of seizures, helping to control or reduce their frequency and intensity.

2. Individualized Treatment Plans:

The choice of medication is not one-size-fits-all. Neurologists tailor treatment plans based on the specific type of seizures, the individual's overall health, and any potential underlying causes. Some medications may be more effective for certain seizure types, while others could exacerbate specific forms of epilepsy.

3. Side Effects and Tolerance:

While epilepsy medications aim to improve the patient's life, they are not without drawbacks. Side effects can range from mild, such as drowsiness or dizziness, to more severe, impacting mood, cognition, or liver function. Striking the right balance between seizure control and manageable side effects is an ongoing challenge, often requiring adjustments in dosage or a switch to an alternative medication.

4. Adherence Challenges:

Successful epilepsy management relies on consistent medication adherence. Skipping doses or abruptly discontinuing medication can lead to breakthrough seizures. Adherence challenges can stem from various factors, including forgetfulness, concerns about side effects, or the financial burden of acquiring the prescribed medications. Healthcare providers play a crucial role in addressing these issues through education, support, and exploring strategies to enhance adherence.

5. Monitoring and Adjustments:
Regular monitoring is essential to assess the effectiveness of the chosen medication and detect any emerging side effects. Neurologists may conduct blood tests to ensure therapeutic drug levels and adjust medication doses accordingly. Frequent communication between patients and healthcare providers is crucial in fine-tuning the treatment plan based on the individual's response.

6. Pregnancy Considerations:
For women with epilepsy who are of childbearing age, the impact of medications extends to pregnancy considerations. Certain antiepileptic drugs may pose risks to the developing fetus. Balancing the need for seizure control with minimizing potential harm to the unborn child requires careful management and consultation with healthcare providers.

7. Exploring Complementary Approaches:

In some cases, individuals may explore complementary or alternative therapies alongside traditional medications. These may include dietary changes, herbal supplements, or lifestyle modifications. While such approaches may complement conventional treatment, it is crucial to consult with healthcare professionals to ensure compatibility and safety.

8. Advances in Medication Research:

The field of epilepsy medication continues to evolve with ongoing research and the development of new drugs. Researchers strive to discover medications with improved efficacy, fewer side effects, and broader applicability across different types of epilepsy. Staying informed about these advancements is essential for both patients and healthcare providers.

Medications are a cornerstone of epilepsy management, offering the potential for seizure control and improved quality of life. However, the impact extends beyond the immediate goal of seizure reduction, encompassing considerations of side effects, adherence challenges, and the ongoing pursuit of optimal treatment strategies. Through a collaborative and individualized approach, healthcare providers and individuals with epilepsy work together to navigate the complex landscape of medication management, striving for a balance that maximizes benefits while minimizing potential drawbacks.

Exploring Alternative Therapies

Alternative therapies offer individuals with epilepsy additional avenues for managing their condition beyond conventional medical approaches. In this chapter, we will delve into the realm of alternative therapies, exploring various methods that have shown promise in complementing traditional treatments and enhancing overall well-being.

1. Mind-Body Practices

Mind-body practices emphasize the connection between mental and physical health, promoting relaxation and stress reduction. Techniques such as yoga and tai chi have gained popularity among individuals with epilepsy. Through controlled movements, deep breathing, and meditation, these practices aim to improve overall mental and physical balance.

Yoga: Incorporating gentle yoga poses can enhance flexibility, balance, and reduce stress. Certain styles, like Hatha or Restorative Yoga, focus on relaxation and mindfulness, potentially aiding in seizure control by mitigating stress triggers.

Tai Chi: This Chinese martial art involves slow, flowing movements and deep breathing. Studies suggest that tai chi may contribute to better seizure management and improved overall quality of life.

2. Dietary Approaches
Diet plays a crucial role in overall health, and some alternative diets have shown promise in managing epilepsy.

Ketogenic Diet: This high-fat, low-carbohydrate diet has been used for decades to control seizures, especially in children with epilepsy. The ketogenic diet induces a state of ketosis, altering the metabolism of the brain and potentially reducing seizure frequency.

Modified Atkins Diet: Similar to the ketogenic diet, the modified Atkins diet is less restrictive in terms of protein intake. It emphasizes a low-carbohydrate and high-fat approach, offering a more feasible option for some individuals.

3. Herbal Supplements
Certain herbs and supplements are believed to have anticonvulsant properties, although scientific evidence supporting their efficacy is limited.

Cannabidiol (CBD): Derived from the cannabis plant, CBD has gained attention for its potential therapeutic effects. Some studies suggest that CBD may help reduce seizure frequency, particularly in certain forms of epilepsy. However, it's essential to note that more research is needed to establish its effectiveness and safety.

Vitamins and Minerals: Some individuals explore the benefits of specific vitamins and minerals, such as vitamin B6, magnesium, and zinc. While these nutrients play essential roles in overall health, their impact on seizure control varies, and it's crucial to approach supplementation under medical guidance.

4. Acupuncture and Acupressure

Rooted in traditional Chinese medicine, acupuncture involves inserting thin needles into specific points on the body to restore balance in the flow of energy, or "qi." Acupressure, a non-invasive alternative, involves applying pressure to these points.

Acupuncture: Limited studies suggest that acupuncture may have a positive impact on seizure frequency and overall well-being. It's essential to consult with a qualified practitioner to ensure safety and efficacy.

Acupressure: While less researched than acupuncture, acupressure may provide relaxation and stress relief. It's a non-invasive option that individuals can explore under the guidance of a knowledgeable practitioner.

5. Biofeedback and Neurofeedback

Biofeedback and neurofeedback involve learning how to control physiological functions using information provided by sensors monitoring various bodily processes.

Biofeedback: This technique helps individuals gain awareness and control over physiological functions like heart rate, muscle tension, and skin temperature. By learning to regulate these functions, some individuals report reduced seizure frequency and improved stress management.

Neurofeedback: Also known as EEG biofeedback, neurofeedback involves training individuals to regulate their brainwave patterns. While research is ongoing, some studies suggest potential benefits in seizure control.

In conclusion, exploring alternative therapies provides individuals with epilepsy a diverse range of options to enhance their well-being. It's crucial to approach these approaches with an open mind, in consultation with healthcare professionals, to ensure a comprehensive and safe approach to epilepsy management. Always remember that individual responses to alternative therapies may vary, and what works for one person may not be suitable for another.

Lifestyle Changes for Seizure Control

Nutrition and Epilepsy

Nutrition plays a crucial role in managing epilepsy, contributing not only to overall well-being but also influencing seizure control. While medication is often a primary component of epilepsy treatment, adopting a balanced and mindful approach to nutrition can enhance the effectiveness of medical interventions. This chapter delves into the intricate relationship between nutrition and epilepsy, exploring dietary strategies that may positively impact seizure management.

Understanding the Link:
The connection between nutrition and epilepsy lies in the intricate balance of chemicals and electrical impulses within the brain. Certain nutrients play key roles in supporting this delicate equilibrium. For instance, omega-3 fatty acids found in fish, flaxseeds, and walnuts contribute to brain health, potentially influencing neurotransmitter function and reducing inflammation. Additionally, vitamins

and minerals like vitamin B6, magnesium, and zinc play essential roles in neurological processes, and their deficiency may exacerbate seizure activity.

The Ketogenic Diet:

One of the most well-known dietary interventions for epilepsy is the ketogenic diet. Originally developed in the 1920s to mimic the biochemical changes associated with fasting, the ketogenic diet is a high-fat, low-carbohydrate, and adequate-protein regimen. The drastic reduction in carbohydrates prompts the body to enter a state of ketosis, where it utilizes ketones as an alternative energy source. This metabolic shift has been shown to reduce seizure frequency, especially in children with refractory epilepsy.

Balanced Nutrition for Seizure Control:

While the ketogenic diet is a specific and often challenging approach, maintaining a balanced and nutritious diet is universally beneficial for individuals with epilepsy. Opting for a variety of whole foods ensures a broad spectrum of essential nutrients. Incorporating fruits, vegetables, whole grains, and lean proteins provides vitamins, minerals, and antioxidants that support overall health and may positively influence seizure thresholds.

Identifying Trigger Foods:
For some individuals with epilepsy, certain foods may act as triggers, potentially influencing seizure occurrence. While triggers vary from person to person, common culprits include caffeine, alcohol, and specific food additives. Keeping a detailed food diary can help identify patterns and potential triggers, enabling individuals to make informed decisions about their diet.

Hydration and Electrolyte Balance:
Maintaining proper hydration is crucial for everyone, but it holds particular significance for those with epilepsy. Dehydration can affect electrolyte balance, potentially triggering seizures. Ensuring an adequate intake of fluids, especially water, helps support overall health and may contribute to seizure prevention.

Supplements and Their Role:
In some cases, nutritional supplements can complement dietary efforts. However, it's essential to consult with healthcare professionals before

incorporating supplements into one's routine. Vitamin and mineral supplements, such as vitamin D and magnesium, may be recommended based on individual nutritional needs and potential deficiencies.

Considerations for Medication Interactions:
Certain foods and supplements can interact with antiepileptic medications, affecting their absorption or effectiveness. Individuals should discuss their diet and any planned supplements with their healthcare team to ensure optimal medication management.

Personalizing Nutrition Strategies:
Nutrition is a highly individualized aspect of epilepsy management. What works for one person may not work for another. Consulting with a registered dietitian or nutritionist experienced in epilepsy care can help tailor dietary recommendations to individual needs, preferences, and health goals.

In conclusion, nutrition plays a multifaceted role in epilepsy management. From the ketogenic diet to maintaining a balanced and varied nutrient intake, individuals with epilepsy can harness the power of nutrition to complement medical interventions. A mindful and individualized approach to nutrition empowers individuals to make informed choices, supporting overall health and potentially contributing to enhanced seizure control.

The Power of Regular Exercise

Regular exercise is a powerful and often underestimated tool in the journey of epilepsy recovery. While it may seem counterintuitive to engage in physical activity when dealing with a condition characterized by unpredictable seizures, numerous studies and anecdotal evidence highlight the positive impact exercise can have on seizure control, overall well-being, and the quality of life for individuals living with epilepsy.

One of the key benefits of regular exercise is its potential to reduce the frequency and severity of seizures. Physical activity has been shown to regulate neurotransmitters in the brain, including serotonin and dopamine, which play crucial roles in mood stabilization and seizure threshold modulation. Additionally, exercise promotes better blood flow and oxygenation to the brain, contributing to a healthier neural environment that may be less prone to seizures.

Engaging in aerobic exercises, such as walking, jogging, swimming, or cycling, has been particularly associated with positive outcomes in epilepsy recovery. These activities increase cardiovascular fitness, improve lung capacity, and enhance overall physical endurance. Beyond the physical benefits, aerobic exercise releases endorphins – the body's natural mood lifters – which can help reduce stress and anxiety, common triggers for seizures.

Strength training exercises, focusing on building muscle mass and endurance, also play a role in epilepsy recovery. Increased muscle tone and strength contribute to better overall body function and coordination, which can be especially beneficial during and after a seizure. Building a strong foundation through resistance training can enhance stability and reduce the risk of injury during seizure episodes.

Yoga, with its combination of physical postures, breath control, and meditation, has gained recognition for its positive effects on epilepsy management. While research is ongoing, some studies suggest that the mindfulness and relaxation components of yoga may help in stress reduction, potentially influencing seizure control. It is crucial, however, to approach yoga under the guidance of a qualified instructor who is aware of your specific condition and can tailor the practice accordingly.

Adopting a regular exercise routine is not only about managing seizures; it also contributes significantly to overall health and well-being. Many individuals with epilepsy face challenges such as weight gain, side effects from medications, and psychological stress. Regular physical activity can address these issues by promoting weight management, improving metabolic health, and positively impacting mental health.

In the context of epilepsy recovery, exercise can serve as a catalyst for building resilience and adapting to the challenges that come with the condition. The discipline required to maintain a consistent exercise routine fosters a sense of control and empowerment, qualities that are invaluable in the face of uncertainty. Developing a routine can also enhance self-esteem and confidence, essential components of a holistic recovery process.

It is essential, however, to approach exercise with caution and consultation with healthcare professionals. Certain activities may pose risks, especially if there is a history of seizures triggered by specific movements or if there are associated health conditions. Personalized advice and guidance can help tailor an exercise plan that maximizes benefits while minimizing potential risks.

In conclusion, the power of regular exercise in epilepsy recovery cannot be overstated. From its impact on seizure control to its broader contributions to physical and mental well-being, exercise emerges as a multifaceted and accessible strategy for those navigating the challenges of epilepsy. Embracing a lifestyle that includes regular physical activity, tailored to individual needs and limitations, can be a transformative step on the path to recovery and improved quality of life.

Stress Management Techniques

Stress management is a crucial aspect of epilepsy recovery, as stress can act as a trigger for seizures in many individuals. Implementing effective stress management techniques not only contributes to seizure control but also enhances overall well-being. In this section, we'll explore various strategies to manage stress in the context of epilepsy recovery.

Mindfulness Meditation:
Mindfulness meditation involves cultivating awareness of the present moment without judgment. This practice has shown promising results in reducing stress levels and improving overall mental health. For individuals recovering from epilepsy, incorporating mindfulness meditation into their daily routine can provide a sense of calm and focus. Techniques such as deep breathing, body scan, and guided meditation can be particularly helpful.

Progressive Muscle Relaxation (PMR):
Progressive Muscle Relaxation is a technique that involves systematically tensing and relaxing different muscle groups in the body. This process helps release physical tension and promotes a state

of relaxation. Regular practice of PMR can contribute to stress reduction and may have a positive impact on seizure management.

Yoga and Tai Chi:
Both yoga and Tai Chi combine physical postures, breathing exercises, and meditation. These mind-body practices not only enhance flexibility and balance but also promote relaxation and stress relief. Incorporating yoga or Tai Chi into an epilepsy recovery plan can contribute to overall well-being, both physically and mentally.

Cognitive Behavioral Therapy (CBT):
CBT is a therapeutic approach that focuses on identifying and changing negative thought patterns and behaviors. For individuals recovering from epilepsy, CBT can help manage stress by addressing anxiety, fear, and other emotional challenges associated with the condition. Learning to reframe thoughts and develop healthier coping mechanisms can be empowering.

Aerobic Exercise:
Regular physical activity has been linked to reduced stress levels and improved mood. Engaging in

aerobic exercises, such as walking, jogging, or swimming, not only promotes physical fitness but also releases endorphins—natural mood lifters. It's essential to choose activities that align with individual fitness levels and preferences.

Relaxation Techniques:
Incorporating relaxation techniques, such as deep breathing exercises and visualization, can be effective in managing stress. Deep breathing, in particular, activates the body's relaxation response, reducing the physiological and psychological impact of stress. Visualization involves creating mental images of peaceful and calming scenes to promote a sense of tranquility.

Journaling:
Writing down thoughts and feelings in a journal can be a therapeutic way to process emotions and manage stress. For those recovering from epilepsy, journaling can provide a constructive outlet for expressing concerns, tracking triggers, and celebrating progress. Reflecting on positive experiences and setting achievable goals can contribute to a more positive mindset.

Time Management:
Effective time management is crucial for stress reduction. Breaking tasks into manageable steps, prioritizing responsibilities, and setting realistic goals can prevent feelings of overwhelm. Creating a structured daily routine can also provide a sense of stability, which is particularly beneficial for individuals navigating the challenges of epilepsy recovery.

Stress management is a vital component of epilepsy recovery. Implementing a combination of mindfulness practices, relaxation techniques, physical activity, and therapeutic approaches like CBT can significantly contribute to stress reduction. It's important for individuals recovering from epilepsy to explore and identify the techniques that work best for them, creating a personalized stress management plan that aligns with their unique needs and preferences. By proactively addressing stress, individuals can not only enhance their overall quality of life but also contribute to better seizure control and long-term well-being.

Building a Support System

Family and Friends as Allies

Family and friends play a pivotal role in the journey of epilepsy recovery, serving as invaluable allies in the pursuit of a healthier and more fulfilling life. Their support, understanding, and encouragement contribute significantly to the overall well-being of individuals grappling with epilepsy. In this exploration, we delve into the multifaceted ways in which family and friends become powerful allies, fostering a sense of community and resilience.

At the heart of the matter is the need for education. Families and friends can act as frontline advocates by educating themselves about epilepsy. Understanding the various types of seizures, triggers, and treatment options empowers them to provide informed and compassionate support. Armed with knowledge, they become better equipped to handle situations, offer assistance during seizures, and make informed decisions in collaboration with healthcare professionals.

Communication emerges as a cornerstone in the allyship between individuals with epilepsy and their loved ones. Open and honest dialogue creates an environment of trust and understanding. Those facing epilepsy often experience a range of emotions, from frustration to anxiety, and having a supportive network allows for the expression of these feelings without judgment. Equally important is the ability of family and friends to express their concerns and feelings, fostering a two-way street of communication that strengthens relationships.

Beyond understanding and communication, practical support is essential. Accompanying a loved one to medical appointments, helping them manage medications, or ensuring a safe environment are tangible ways in which family and friends can actively contribute to epilepsy management. Recognizing potential triggers and collaborating with individuals to develop strategies for daily living are crucial aspects of this hands-on support. This involvement not only aids in seizure prevention but also reinforces the sense of solidarity in the face of epilepsy-related challenges.

Social stigma surrounding epilepsy persists, making the role of allies even more critical. Families and friends can act as advocates, dispelling myths and misconceptions about epilepsy within their social circles. By openly discussing the condition and sharing accurate information, they contribute to a more inclusive and empathetic community, reducing the isolation often felt by those with epilepsy.

Patience emerges as a virtue in the allyship dynamic. Epilepsy can be unpredictable, and its management may require adjustments over time. Family and friends who approach the journey with patience help create a supportive environment where individuals with epilepsy feel accepted and understood. This patience extends to the learning curve associated with managing seizures and adapting to lifestyle changes, fostering a sense of resilience within the support network.

In times of crisis, the strength of familial and friendly bonds truly shines. During seizures, the immediate assistance of a family member or friend can be a lifeline. Knowing how to respond appropriately and confidently can make a significant difference in minimizing risks and ensuring the well-being of the individual with epilepsy. Training in basic first aid for seizures becomes an essential aspect of allyship, emphasizing the importance of quick and effective action.

As the journey of epilepsy recovery unfolds, the emotional well-being of both individuals with epilepsy and their allies becomes intertwined. Family and friends often witness the resilience, courage, and determination displayed by their loved ones facing epilepsy. In turn, these individuals draw strength from the unwavering support provided by their allies. This reciprocal relationship creates a foundation of emotional support that contributes to the overall mental health and quality of life for everyone involved.

In conclusion, the alliance between individuals with epilepsy and their family and friends is a powerful force in the pursuit of recovery. From education and communication to practical assistance and emotional support, the role of allies is multifaceted. As they navigate the challenges and triumphs together, this collective effort not only aids in epilepsy management but also fosters a sense of community, understanding, and resilience that transcends the boundaries of the condition. Family and friends, as allies, become not just a support system but a source of strength, unity, and hope in the journey toward a brighter, epilepsy-aware future.

Communicating with Healthcare Providers

Effective communication with healthcare providers is paramount in managing and recovering from epilepsy. Establishing a strong and open line of communication ensures that you receive the best possible care and empowers you to actively participate in decisions about your health. In this section, we'll explore key aspects of communicating with healthcare providers, fostering a collaborative relationship that promotes your well-being.

Building a Foundation of Trust

Trust is the cornerstone of any successful relationship, and the one between a patient and their healthcare provider is no exception. Building trust involves open and honest communication. Share your complete medical history, including any previous experiences with seizures, treatments, and medications. This information equips your healthcare provider with essential context to tailor their recommendations to your unique situation.

Active Participation in Conversations

Being an active participant in conversations with your healthcare provider is vital. Prepare for appointments by jotting down questions or concerns beforehand. Discuss your symptoms, triggers, and any lifestyle changes you've noticed. This collaborative approach helps your healthcare provider gain a comprehensive understanding of your condition.

Ask questions about your diagnosis, treatment options, and potential side effects of medications. Understanding the rationale behind recommendations empowers you to make informed decisions about your care. If there are uncertainties, don't hesitate to seek clarification—effective communication requires a shared understanding between you and your healthcare team.

Shared Decision-Making

Engage in shared decision-making with your healthcare provider to determine the best course of action for your epilepsy management. Express your preferences, values, and goals, and work collaboratively to create a treatment plan that aligns with them. This shared approach not only fosters a sense of ownership over your healthcare journey but also increases adherence to the agreed-upon plan.

Regular Follow-Up and Progress Updates

Maintaining an ongoing dialogue with your healthcare provider through regular follow-up appointments is crucial. These sessions provide an opportunity to discuss your progress, address concerns, and make any necessary adjustments to your treatment plan. If you experience changes in your symptoms or lifestyle, communicate these developments promptly to ensure timely interventions.

Reporting Medication Side Effects

Communication extends beyond the exchange of information—it also involves reporting any side effects or concerns related to your medications. If you experience adverse reactions, share them with your healthcare provider promptly. They can then explore alternative medications or adjust dosages to minimize side effects while maintaining effective seizure control.

Emergency Communication Plan

Developing an emergency communication plan is essential, especially in the context of epilepsy. Work with your healthcare provider to create a clear and concise plan outlining what steps to take during a seizure or if there are unexpected complications. Share this plan with family members, close friends, and colleagues to ensure a coordinated response in case of emergencies.

Utilizing Technology for Communication

In today's digital age, technology can enhance communication between patients and healthcare providers. Utilize patient portals, email, or secure messaging systems offered by healthcare facilities to share non-urgent updates, ask questions, or request prescription refills. Embrace these tools to streamline communication and stay connected between appointments.

Advocating for Yourself

Effective communication also involves advocating for your needs. If you feel that your concerns are not adequately addressed or if you seek a second opinion, express these desires openly. Your active involvement in your healthcare journey is a key driver of positive outcomes.

Communication with healthcare providers is a dynamic and collaborative process that forms the bedrock of effective epilepsy management. Establishing trust, actively participating in conversations, engaging in shared decision-making, and utilizing technology are integral components of this process. By fostering open communication, you not only enhance the quality of care you receive but also play an active role in your journey towards epilepsy recovery. Remember, your voice matters, and your healthcare team is there to support and collaborate with you every step of the way.

Joining Epilepsy Support Groups

Joining epilepsy support groups can be a transformative and empowering experience for individuals navigating the challenges of epilepsy. These groups provide a valuable platform for connecting with others who share similar experiences, offering a sense of community, understanding, and encouragement. In this journey towards recovery, the camaraderie found within epilepsy support groups becomes a crucial pillar of support.

1. The Power of Shared Experiences:
One of the most significant advantages of joining an epilepsy support group is the opportunity to share experiences with individuals facing similar challenges. Epilepsy can be a complex condition with various manifestations, and each person's journey is unique. Engaging with a support group allows individuals to express their thoughts, fears, and triumphs in a space where others can relate on a deep and personal level. This shared understanding creates a sense of belonging and reduces the isolation that individuals with epilepsy might often feel.

2. Emotional Support and Empathy:

Living with epilepsy can be emotionally taxing, affecting not only the individual but also their loved ones. Support groups provide a safe space to express emotions openly, whether it's frustration, fear, or even moments of joy and achievement. Fellow group members can offer empathy and understanding, providing emotional support that goes beyond what friends and family might comprehend. This shared emotional journey fosters a strong sense of solidarity among group participants.

3. Practical Advice and Coping Strategies:

Navigating the practical aspects of life with epilepsy often involves learning effective coping strategies. Support groups become a treasure trove of practical advice, as members share their strategies for managing medication side effects, handling disclosure in the workplace, or dealing with the challenges of daily life. This collective wisdom can significantly enhance an individual's ability to cope with the various facets of epilepsy and its impact on day-to-day living.

4. Education and Awareness:

Epilepsy support groups also serve as educational platforms. Through discussions, presentations, and shared resources, participants can deepen their understanding of epilepsy, its treatments, and the latest advancements in the field. This knowledge not only empowers individuals in managing their condition but also contributes to raising awareness within the broader community. Education becomes a tool for dispelling myths and reducing the stigma associated with epilepsy.

5. A Sense of Community:

Building a sense of community is at the heart of epilepsy support groups. Knowing that there are others who understand the challenges and victories of living with epilepsy creates a supportive environment. This community extends beyond the confines of support group meetings, often leading to lasting friendships. The bond formed through shared experiences becomes a powerful force in overcoming the feelings of isolation that epilepsy can sometimes impose.

6. Advocacy and Collective Action:

Epilepsy support groups often evolve into advocates for change and awareness. The collective voice of individuals who have experienced the impact of epilepsy firsthand can be a powerful catalyst for societal change. Whether it involves advocating for better healthcare policies, increased research funding, or improved workplace accommodations, the unity found in support groups can drive meaningful change.

7. Motivation and Inspiration:
Witnessing the triumphs of others in the face of epilepsy can be incredibly motivating. Support group participants share success stories, illustrating that it is possible to lead fulfilling lives despite the challenges posed by epilepsy. These narratives serve as beacons of hope, inspiring individuals to set and achieve their own goals, fostering a positive and determined mindset.

In conclusion, joining epilepsy support groups is not just about finding solace; it's about forging connections that have the power to transform lives. From shared experiences and emotional support to practical advice and advocacy, these groups provide a holistic approach to navigating the complex landscape of epilepsy. The sense of community formed within these groups becomes a beacon of strength, guiding individuals towards a more empowered and resilient life beyond epilepsy.

Empowering Your Mind

Mindfulness and Meditation

Mindfulness and meditation have become integral components of holistic well-being, offering individuals profound tools to navigate the complexities of modern life. Rooted in ancient contemplative practices, these techniques have transcended cultural boundaries to find a place in diverse societies worldwide. In the pursuit of mental and emotional balance, mindfulness and meditation offer a sanctuary for self-discovery and personal growth.

At its essence, mindfulness involves cultivating an acute awareness of the present moment. It's the art of being fully engaged in the here and now, without judgment. This practice encourages individuals to observe their thoughts and feelings with a non-reactive mindset, fostering a deeper understanding of their inner landscape. Meditation, on the other hand, is a structured exercise aimed at achieving a heightened state of awareness, often through focused attention or guided visualization.

One of the primary benefits of mindfulness and meditation lies in their ability to mitigate stress and promote relaxation. In a fast-paced world filled with constant stimuli, individuals frequently find themselves overwhelmed by the demands of daily life. Mindfulness offers a sanctuary, a mental space where one can detach from stressors and regain a sense of calm. The practice encourages intentional breathing and a gentle redirection of attention, allowing individuals to create a buffer against the chaos of their surroundings.

Moreover, mindfulness and meditation have been scientifically proven to positively impact mental health. Research indicates that regular practice can reduce symptoms of anxiety and depression. By fostering an awareness of thoughts and emotions without attachment, individuals gain a newfound resilience in the face of life's challenges. The simple act of observing one's thoughts can break the cycle of rumination, providing a fresh perspective and paving the way for healthier mental patterns.

In the realm of physical well-being, mindfulness and meditation exhibit remarkable effects. Studies suggest that these practices can contribute to lower blood pressure, improved immune function, and enhanced overall cardiovascular health. The mind-body connection is a powerful force, and as individuals cultivate mindfulness, they often find themselves more attuned to the needs of their bodies, making conscious choices that promote well-being.

The cognitive benefits of mindfulness and meditation are equally compelling. These practices have been linked to improved concentration and heightened cognitive function. By training the mind to focus on the present moment, individuals develop a mental discipline that extends beyond the meditation session. This enhanced cognitive control can positively impact various aspects of life, from work performance to academic achievement.

Mindfulness and meditation also play a transformative role in relationships. As individuals become more attuned to their own thoughts and emotions, they naturally develop a heightened sense of empathy and compassion. This increased emotional intelligence fosters deeper connections with others, as individuals learn to approach relationships with an open heart and a non-judgmental mindset.

Practical integration of mindfulness and meditation into daily life is essential for realizing their full potential. Creating a dedicated space and time for these practices allows individuals to establish consistency, making them more accessible during moments of stress. Whether through guided meditations, mindful breathing exercises, or silent contemplation, the key lies in making these practices a personal ritual that aligns with individual preferences and schedules.

In conclusion, mindfulness and meditation offer a profound journey inward, unlocking the potential for self-discovery, resilience, and overall well-being. These ancient practices, now backed by modern science, provide a timeless refuge in a rapidly changing world. By embracing the art of being present, individuals can cultivate a rich inner life that positively ripples into every facet of their existence, fostering a holistic and transformative approach to living.

Cognitive Behavioral Strategies

Cognitive Behavioral Strategies (CBS) play a pivotal role in empowering individuals on their journey towards epilepsy recovery. Rooted in the idea that our thoughts, feelings, and behaviors are interconnected, CBS focuses on identifying and modifying negative patterns of thinking to promote positive outcomes. In the context of epilepsy, these strategies offer valuable tools for managing stress, anxiety, and improving overall well-being.

Understanding Cognitive Behavioral Strategies

At its core, Cognitive Behavioral Therapy (CBT) targets the cognitive processes that contribute to emotional distress and behavioral challenges. For individuals with epilepsy, the impact of seizures can extend beyond the physical realm, influencing mental and emotional aspects of their lives. CBS aims to address and reframe these cognitive patterns, fostering resilience and enhancing the ability to cope with the challenges associated with epilepsy.

Restructuring Negative Thought Patterns

One key component of CBS involves recognizing and challenging negative thought patterns.

Individuals with epilepsy may grapple with feelings of fear, helplessness, or anxiety related to their condition. Through cognitive restructuring, individuals learn to identify automatic negative thoughts and replace them with more balanced, realistic perspectives.

For example, someone experiencing anxiety about the possibility of a seizure in a public place might initially think, "I can't go out; I might have a seizure and embarrass myself." Through CBS, they can challenge this thought by considering evidence to the contrary, such as past experiences of successfully managing outings without seizures. This process helps shift the mindset from avoidance to empowerment.

Behavior Modification Techniques
In conjunction with cognitive restructuring, CBS incorporates behavior modification techniques. This involves identifying behaviors associated with negative thoughts and developing strategies to modify or replace them with more adaptive alternatives. For individuals with epilepsy, this could involve addressing avoidance behaviors, such as

refraining from social activities due to fear of having a seizure.

Gradual exposure, a common behavioral technique, encourages individuals to face feared situations in a controlled and systematic manner. This helps build confidence and resilience over time. A person might start by engaging in small, manageable social interactions and gradually progress to more challenging situations, all while implementing cognitive strategies to manage anxiety.

Stress Management and Relaxation Techniques
Given the potential stressors associated with epilepsy, stress management is a crucial aspect of CBS. Learning relaxation techniques, such as deep breathing, progressive muscle relaxation, or guided imagery, can significantly reduce stress levels. These techniques not only contribute to overall well-being but also serve as effective coping mechanisms during or after seizures.

In the context of epilepsy recovery, stress management becomes an essential skill. Individuals may encounter stressors related to medication side effects, uncertainty about seizure triggers, or concerns about societal perceptions. CBS equips individuals with practical tools to navigate and mitigate these stressors, promoting a more adaptive response to life's challenges.

Goal Setting and Positive Reinforcement

Setting realistic and achievable goals is another cornerstone of CBS. Individuals with epilepsy may face unique challenges, but goal setting provides a roadmap for progress. Whether it's improving medication adherence, increasing physical activity, or enhancing social engagement, establishing clear and attainable goals creates a sense of purpose and direction.

Positive reinforcement plays a crucial role in maintaining motivation and sustaining behavioral changes. Acknowledging and celebrating small victories, no matter how seemingly insignificant, contributes to a positive feedback loop. This process encourages continued effort and resilience in the face of setbacks, fostering a proactive approach to epilepsy management.

Integrating Cognitive Behavioral Strategies into Daily Life

The effectiveness of Cognitive Behavioral Strategies lies in their integration into daily life. Consistent practice of cognitive restructuring, behavior modification, stress management, and goal setting transforms these strategies from theoretical concepts to practical tools for navigating the challenges of epilepsy.

In conclusion, Cognitive Behavioral Strategies offer a holistic approach to epilepsy recovery by addressing the interconnected relationship between thoughts, feelings, and behaviors. By empowering individuals to reframe negative thought patterns, modify maladaptive behaviors, and cultivate stress management skills, CBS becomes a powerful ally in the journey towards enhanced well-being and resilience in the face of epilepsy.

Goal Setting for Recovery

In the realm of epilepsy recovery, setting meaningful and achievable goals is not merely a task but a powerful strategy for empowerment and progress. As individuals navigate the challenges of living with epilepsy, establishing clear objectives can serve as a guiding light toward a more fulfilling and resilient life.

The Foundation of Goal Setting

At its core, goal setting is about identifying specific, measurable, achievable, relevant, and time-bound (SMART) objectives. For someone on the path to epilepsy recovery, these goals extend beyond mere health outcomes; they encompass physical, emotional, and social well-being. By establishing a foundation of well-defined goals, individuals can create a roadmap that not only addresses their medical needs but also enriches their overall quality of life.

Personalizing Your Journey

One size does not fit all when it comes to epilepsy recovery. Each person's experience is unique, influenced by various factors such as seizure types, medications, and lifestyle. Therefore, the first step in goal setting is self-reflection. Understand your strengths, acknowledge your limitations, and recognize the aspects of life that bring you joy and fulfillment.

Consider breaking down your goals into different domains: health, relationships, career, and personal growth. This holistic approach allows for a comprehensive exploration of what truly matters to you and what steps are needed for a well-rounded recovery.

Short-Term Wins and Long-Term Aspirations
In the journey of epilepsy recovery, celebrating small victories is as crucial as pursuing long-term aspirations. Short-term goals provide a sense of achievement, boosting motivation and confidence. These could be daily exercises, consistent medication routines, or adopting stress-management techniques.

Simultaneously, long-term goals act as a beacon, guiding individuals towards their overarching vision of recovery. This could include achieving seizure control, successfully managing triggers, or even exploring new career opportunities. Balancing short-term wins with long-term aspirations creates a dynamic synergy that propels one forward on the road to recovery.

The Power of Positive Framing

Epilepsy recovery is not solely about overcoming challenges but also about embracing possibilities. Framing goals in a positive light fosters a mindset of resilience and optimism. For instance, rather than focusing on avoiding triggers, set goals that involve incorporating positive habits. This might include establishing a consistent sleep routine or engaging in activities that promote emotional well-being.

Positive framing extends to the language used in goal setting. Instead of stating what you want to avoid, express your goals in affirmative terms. For example, shift from "reduce stress" to "incorporate stress-reducing activities daily." This shift in language reinforces the proactive nature of your journey.

Goal Setting as a Collaborative Process

While personal aspirations are paramount, involving healthcare professionals, family, and friends in the goal-setting process can be immensely beneficial. Healthcare providers can offer insights into setting realistic health-related goals, ensuring they align with your treatment plan. Friends and family provide essential support and encouragement, transforming the journey into a collective effort.

Communication is key. Clearly articulate your goals to your support network, fostering understanding and collaboration. Regular check-ins with healthcare providers and loved ones not only track progress but also create a sense of accountability, enhancing commitment to the recovery journey.

Adapting to Change
Flexibility is inherent in the recovery process. Unexpected challenges may arise, requiring adjustments to your goals. Embracing adaptability is not a sign of failure but a testament to your resilience. Be open to refining your goals based on evolving circumstances, and recognize that progress is often nonlinear.

Goal setting is not a rigid process but a dynamic and empowering tool in the arsenal of epilepsy recovery. It transforms the journey into a purposeful expedition, providing direction and motivation. As you navigate the path to recovery, remember that your goals are not mere destinations but beacons guiding you toward a life filled with purpose, resilience, and fulfillment.

Overcoming Challenges

Navigating Stigma

Navigating the complex terrain of stigma is an integral part of the epilepsy recovery journey. While medical advancements have provided a better understanding of the condition, societal misconceptions and stereotypes still cast shadows on those living with epilepsy. This chapter delves into the multifaceted aspects of navigating stigma, offering insights, strategies, and empowerment for individuals seeking to overcome the challenges associated with public perception.

Understanding Stigma:
Stigma surrounding epilepsy often stems from a lack of awareness and outdated beliefs. Historically, epilepsy has been shrouded in myths associating it with supernatural forces or erratic behavior. These misconceptions contribute to the stigma that individuals with epilepsy face, impacting various facets of their lives, including personal relationships, employment opportunities, and self-esteem.

Educating Others:

One powerful strategy for combating stigma is education. Individuals with epilepsy, their families, and healthcare providers play pivotal roles in dispelling myths and fostering understanding. Public awareness campaigns, school programs, and community outreach initiatives can contribute to dismantling stereotypes and creating an environment where epilepsy is viewed through an informed lens.

Empowering Self-Advocacy:

Navigating stigma often involves empowering individuals with epilepsy to become advocates for themselves. This may involve open communication about the condition, sharing personal stories, and correcting misconceptions. By taking an active role in educating others, individuals with epilepsy can contribute to breaking down the barriers of misunderstanding that fuel stigma.

Challenges in Personal Relationships:

Stigma can manifest within personal relationships, impacting friendships, romantic partnerships, and familial connections. Fear and ignorance may lead to strained interactions, making it essential for individuals with epilepsy to engage in open and honest conversations with their loved ones. Building a support network that understands epilepsy and is willing to learn fosters an environment of empathy and acceptance.

The Workplace and Epilepsy:

The professional sphere is not immune to the challenges of stigma. Individuals with epilepsy may encounter discrimination in the workplace due to misconceptions about their abilities and reliability. To navigate these challenges, it is crucial to be informed about workplace rights, engage in dialogue with employers, and seek accommodations when necessary. Creating an atmosphere of open communication helps dispel preconceived notions and fosters a more inclusive work environment.

Coping with Emotional Struggles:

Stigma doesn't only manifest externally but can also take a toll on an individual's emotional well-being. Coping with the emotional aspects of stigma involves developing resilience and a positive mindset. Support groups, therapy, and mindfulness practices can be invaluable tools for managing the emotional impact of societal judgment.

Celebrating Diversity:

An essential aspect of navigating stigma is promoting a celebration of diversity within the epilepsy community. Every individual's experience with epilepsy is unique, and acknowledging this diversity helps challenge stereotypical views. By showcasing the accomplishments and capabilities of those with epilepsy, the community can contribute to reshaping public perceptions.

Legal Protections and Advocacy:

Understanding and utilizing legal protections against discrimination is a crucial aspect of navigating stigma. Many countries have laws in place to safeguard individuals with disabilities, including epilepsy. Advocacy for these rights, both individually and collectively, contributes to the ongoing battle against discriminatory practices.

Moving Forward with Confidence:

Navigating stigma is an ongoing process that requires resilience, education, and a collective effort. By addressing stigma head-on, individuals with epilepsy can reclaim control over their narrative and contribute to a more inclusive and understanding society. Through education, self-advocacy, and fostering supportive communities, the epilepsy recovery journey becomes not just a personal triumph but a catalyst for positive change on a broader scale.

Coping with Emotional Struggles

Coping with emotional struggles is a vital aspect of navigating the challenging terrain of epilepsy. The emotional toll that accompanies a chronic condition like epilepsy can be profound, affecting not only the individual diagnosed but also their loved ones. In this chapter, we delve into various strategies and insights to help you effectively manage and cope with the emotional aspects of living with epilepsy.

Understanding the Emotional Impact:
Epilepsy can evoke a range of emotions, including fear, frustration, anxiety, and even depression. The uncertainty of when a seizure might occur, concerns about social stigma, and the impact on daily life can contribute to emotional distress. It's essential to acknowledge and understand these emotions as a crucial first step in coping.

Seeking Professional Support:
One of the most effective ways to cope with emotional struggles is by seeking professional support. Mental health professionals, such as psychologists or counselors, can provide a safe space to express your feelings and develop coping mechanisms. Therapy can help you explore the emotional impact of epilepsy, address any underlying issues, and build resilience.

Building a Support System:
Surrounding yourself with a supportive network of friends and family is instrumental in coping with emotional struggles. Share your experiences, educate those close to you about epilepsy, and let them be a source of understanding and encouragement. A strong support system can offer comfort during challenging times and celebrate your victories, both big and small.

Educating Yourself and Others:
Knowledge is empowering. Understanding epilepsy, its triggers, and how to respond during a seizure can help alleviate anxiety. Similarly, educating those around you can dispel myths and reduce the stigma associated with the condition. A well-informed

community is more likely to provide the understanding and support needed to cope with emotional challenges.

Developing Coping Mechanisms:
Identify and cultivate healthy coping mechanisms that work for you. This might include mindfulness practices, such as meditation or deep breathing exercises, to manage stress. Engaging in hobbies, physical activity, or creative pursuits can also serve as effective outlets for emotional expression and stress relief.

Setting Realistic Expectations:
Living with epilepsy may require adjusting expectations, both for yourself and others. Recognize your limitations while also acknowledging your strengths. Setting realistic goals and celebrating achievements, no matter how small, can contribute to a positive mindset and improved emotional well-being.

Addressing Social Stigma:
Social stigma remains a significant challenge for individuals with epilepsy. Addressing misconceptions head-on, advocating for yourself,

and educating others can help break down barriers. Remember that epilepsy does not define you, and challenging societal norms can contribute to a more supportive and understanding environment.

Connecting with Peers:
Joining epilepsy support groups or connecting with individuals who share similar experiences can provide a sense of community and understanding. Sharing stories, tips, and coping strategies with peers who've faced similar emotional struggles can be both validating and empowering.

Monitoring and Managing Medication Side Effects:
Some antiepileptic medications may have emotional side effects. It's crucial to communicate openly with your healthcare provider about any changes in mood or emotional well-being. Adjustments to medication or additional support, such as counseling, may be necessary to manage these side effects effectively.

Celebrating Successes:
Amidst the challenges, take time to acknowledge and celebrate your successes. Whether it's achieving a personal goal, managing stress more effectively, or

simply navigating a particularly difficult day, recognizing and celebrating your triumphs can bolster your emotional resilience.

Coping with emotional struggles in the context of epilepsy requires a multi-faceted approach. From seeking professional support to building a robust support system, educating yourself and others, and developing healthy coping mechanisms, there are numerous strategies to enhance emotional well-being. Remember that it's okay to seek help, and by actively addressing the emotional aspects of epilepsy, you pave the way for a more fulfilling and resilient life.

Facing Employment and Social Hurdles

Navigating the realms of employment and social interactions can pose unique challenges for individuals living with epilepsy. In this chapter, we delve into the multifaceted aspects of facing employment and social hurdles, shedding light on the obstacles encountered and offering strategies for overcoming them.

Understanding Employment Challenges:
Securing and maintaining employment can be particularly challenging for individuals with epilepsy. Employers may harbor misconceptions about the condition, leading to biases and stigmatization. Concerns about potential seizures at the workplace often contribute to a hesitancy in hiring individuals with epilepsy. Moreover, the fear of legal liabilities can cast a shadow on the hiring process.

To overcome these challenges, it is crucial to foster open communication between employees and employers. Individuals with epilepsy should feel empowered to disclose their condition in a supportive and understanding environment. Employers, on the other hand, benefit from education about epilepsy, dispelling myths and fostering a workplace culture that values diversity and inclusivity.

Navigating Social Stigma:
Social stigma remains a pervasive issue for those living with epilepsy. Misconceptions and fear surrounding seizures can lead to isolation and discrimination. Building awareness within communities is essential to dispel myths and foster an environment of acceptance.

Creating platforms for open dialogue can help break down barriers. Individuals with epilepsy can share their experiences, helping others understand the condition better. Emphasizing that epilepsy does not define a person's capabilities is a powerful way to challenge societal stereotypes.

Embracing Accommodations:
In the workplace, reasonable accommodations can play a pivotal role in ensuring equal opportunities for individuals with epilepsy. Flexibility in work hours, consideration for medical appointments, and providing a safe and quiet space can significantly contribute to a conducive work environment.

Educating employers about the minimal impact these accommodations have on overall productivity is essential. Many individuals with epilepsy lead successful, fulfilling professional lives with the right support and understanding from their workplaces.

Overcoming Employment Discrimination:
Legislation plays a crucial role in protecting the rights of individuals with epilepsy in the workplace. Understanding and advocating for these rights is key to overcoming discriminatory practices. The Americans with Disabilities Act (ADA) in the United States, for instance, prohibits discrimination based on disability, ensuring equal opportunities for employment.

Being proactive in seeking legal advice and understanding one's rights can empower individuals to challenge discriminatory practices. Additionally, fostering alliances with advocacy groups can provide a collective voice against employment discrimination.

Building a Supportive Social Network:
Social interactions can be a source of strength and resilience for individuals with epilepsy. However, the fear of judgment may lead to social withdrawal. Establishing a strong support network of friends and

family can provide the emotional foundation needed to navigate social hurdles.

Engaging in epilepsy support groups allows individuals to connect with others facing similar challenges. These groups offer a platform for shared experiences, advice, and encouragement. Knowing that one is not alone in their journey can boost confidence and combat the isolation that social stigma can impose.

Educating the Community:
Community education is a powerful tool for dispelling myths and fostering inclusivity. Workshops, seminars, and awareness campaigns can contribute to changing attitudes toward epilepsy. By highlighting the capabilities of individuals living with epilepsy and emphasizing their contributions to society, community perceptions can shift positively.

Empowering individuals with epilepsy to share their stories in public forums can humanize the condition, challenging stereotypes and fostering empathy within the community. Education is a collective effort that involves individuals, communities, and organizations working together to create a more inclusive and understanding society.

In conclusion, facing employment and social hurdles as an individual with epilepsy requires a multifaceted approach. Open communication, education, legal awareness, and building supportive networks all play crucial roles in overcoming these challenges. By fostering understanding and inclusivity, we can work towards a society where individuals with epilepsy are not defined by their condition but celebrated for their unique strengths and contributions.

Seizure Safety and First Aid

Creating a Safe Environment

Living with epilepsy necessitates creating a safe and supportive environment that minimizes potential risks and enhances overall well-being. The journey to achieving this safety involves a combination of practical adjustments, education, and fostering understanding among those sharing the same space.

Minimizing Triggers: One of the first steps in crafting a safe environment for individuals with epilepsy involves identifying and minimizing potential triggers. While triggers can vary widely among individuals, common factors include lack of sleep, stress, and certain sensory stimuli. By understanding personal triggers, one can take proactive measures to avoid or manage them effectively.

Home Modifications: Adapting the home environment to reduce seizure risks is crucial. This may involve simple changes such as securing sharp objects, padding hard surfaces, and installing safety gates for stairs. Additionally, ensuring that living spaces are well-lit and clutter-free can prevent accidental falls during seizures.

Seizure Response Plans: Developing a comprehensive seizure response plan is fundamental for both the person with epilepsy and those around them. This plan should outline specific actions to take during a seizure, including how to provide first aid, when to seek medical attention, and whom to contact for support. Educating family members, friends, and colleagues about this plan fosters a sense of preparedness and confidence in handling seizure-related situations.

Medical Identification: Wearing a medical identification bracelet or necklace is a small yet impactful measure that can communicate critical information to bystanders or emergency responders in the event of a seizure. This simple accessory can convey details about the individual's condition, prescribed medications, and emergency contacts, facilitating timely and appropriate care.

Navigating Social Hurdles Associated with Epilepsy
While creating a safe physical environment is vital, individuals with epilepsy often encounter social challenges that require resilience, open communication, and community understanding.

Stigma and Misconceptions: Epilepsy is still surrounded by misconceptions and stigmas that can affect social interactions. Overcoming these hurdles involves raising awareness and promoting accurate information about the condition. Open conversations, educational initiatives, and personal storytelling play pivotal roles in dismantling stereotypes and fostering an inclusive environment.

Employment Challenges: Individuals with epilepsy may face unique challenges in the workplace, ranging from concerns about disclosure to the fear of discrimination. Creating a supportive work environment involves proactive communication with employers and colleagues. Employers can benefit from understanding the nature of epilepsy, implementing reasonable accommodations, and fostering an atmosphere of inclusivity.

Social Isolation: The fear of having a seizure in public can contribute to social isolation. Building a strong support system, both online and offline, can counteract feelings of loneliness. Engaging with epilepsy support groups, where individuals can share experiences and strategies, can be particularly beneficial. Additionally, friends and family members can play a crucial role in creating a supportive and inclusive social environment.

Educational Advocacy: For individuals navigating the education system, advocating for one's needs is essential. This may involve working with teachers, school administrators, and special education professionals to implement necessary accommodations and ensure a positive learning experience. By fostering understanding and cooperation within educational institutions, students with epilepsy can thrive academically and socially.

In conclusion, creating a safe environment for epilepsy management encompasses both physical adjustments and social considerations. By identifying and minimizing triggers, adapting living spaces, and educating those in close proximity, individuals with epilepsy can enhance their overall well-being. Simultaneously, addressing social hurdles through awareness, open communication, and community support can contribute to a more inclusive and understanding society for those living with epilepsy.

First Aid Tips for Seizures

In times of a seizure, having a solid understanding of first aid can make a significant difference in ensuring the safety and well-being of the individual experiencing the episode. Seizures, whether due to epilepsy or other causes, can be distressing for both the person having the seizure and those witnessing it. Here are essential first aid tips for seizures:

1. Stay Calm and Assess the Situation:
When witnessing a seizure, it's crucial to stay calm. Panic can escalate the situation and hinder your ability to provide effective assistance. Take a deep breath, and observe the person having the seizure. Assess the surroundings to identify any potential hazards.

2. Time the Duration:

Keep track of the seizure's duration. While seizures can feel prolonged, they typically last for a short period. If a seizure lasts longer than five minutes or if another seizure immediately follows, it's a medical emergency, and you should call for professional help immediately.

3. Ensure a Safe Environment:

Create a safe space by moving sharp or harmful objects away from the person. Remove glasses and any tight clothing around the neck to prevent injury. Cushion the person's head with a soft object to minimize the risk of head injuries.

4. Do Not Restrain:

Avoid restraining the person during a seizure. Allow the seizure to run its course naturally. Restraining can lead to injury or increased distress for the individual.

5. Turn to the Side:

Gently turn the person onto their side to help keep the airway clear. This can prevent saliva or vomit from causing choking. Place them in a recovery position, supporting their head with a soft object and ensuring their breathing is unobstructed.

6. Time the Seizure:
Continue to time the duration of the seizure. If it exceeds five minutes or if there are repeated seizures without recovery in between, seek emergency medical attention by calling for an ambulance.

7. Comfort and Reassure:
While the person may not be fully aware during the seizure, offering comfort and reassurance afterward can be beneficial. Speak calmly and reassuringly, helping them understand what happened and that they are safe.

8. Monitor Breathing:
Pay close attention to the person's breathing. If they experience difficulty breathing after the seizure, consider providing basic life support measures such as CPR. However, it's crucial to be trained in CPR techniques before attempting them.

9. Be Aware of Postictal State:
After the seizure ends, the person may enter a postictal state characterized by confusion, fatigue, or

sleepiness. Allow them to rest and recover, and be patient as they regain awareness. Provide assistance as needed but avoid overwhelming them with stimuli.

10. Seek Medical Attention:

If it's the person's first seizure, or if there are any concerns about their well-being, seek medical attention. Consult with a healthcare professional to determine the cause of the seizure and establish an appropriate course of action.

In summary, first aid for seizures involves staying calm, ensuring a safe environment, and providing support without restraint. Monitoring the duration, turning the person to their side, and seeking medical attention when necessary are essential components of effective seizure first aid. By being prepared and informed, individuals can contribute to a safer and more supportive experience for someone going through a seizure.

Flourishing Beyond Epilepsy

Embracing a Positive Mindset

Embracing a Positive Mindset in the face of epilepsy is not just a philosophical approach; it's a powerful tool for navigating the challenges of this condition and fostering overall well-being. In a journey marked by uncertainty, positivity becomes a guiding force, shaping perceptions, influencing choices, and laying the foundation for resilience.

One of the fundamental aspects of cultivating a positive mindset is reframing. Individuals with epilepsy often grapple with feelings of frustration, fear, and helplessness. By reframing challenges as opportunities for growth, learning, and adaptation, a positive mindset can transform adversity into a catalyst for personal development. This shift in perspective allows individuals to focus on their strengths, resilience, and capacity to overcome obstacles.

Mindfulness, another cornerstone of positivity, plays a crucial role in epilepsy recovery. The practice of being fully present in the moment enables individuals to detach from the anxieties about past seizures or worries about future ones. Mindfulness encourages a non-judgmental awareness of one's thoughts and feelings, fostering self-compassion and reducing the emotional burden that often accompanies epilepsy.

Furthermore, gratitude emerges as a potent force in fostering a positive mindset. Despite the challenges posed by epilepsy, acknowledging and appreciating the aspects of life that bring joy and fulfillment can be transformative. Gratitude shifts the focus from what may be lacking to what is present, promoting a sense of abundance and resilience in the face of adversity.

A positive mindset also involves setting and pursuing realistic goals. Whether they are related to managing seizure triggers, adopting a healthier lifestyle, or achieving personal aspirations, setting and attaining goals provides a sense of purpose and accomplishment. Small victories contribute to an overall positive outlook, reinforcing the belief in one's ability to navigate the complexities of epilepsy.

Social support is a vital component of embracing a positive mindset. Building a network of understanding family and friends, connecting with support groups, and sharing experiences with others facing similar challenges can be empowering. The exchange of support and encouragement fosters a sense of community, diminishing feelings of isolation and contributing to a more positive emotional state.

Challenges may persist, but a positive mindset helps individuals view setbacks as temporary and surmountable. It encourages a proactive approach to problem-solving and resilience-building, recognizing that setbacks are not indicators of failure but rather opportunities for refinement and growth. This mindset instills a belief in one's ability to adapt, learn, and move forward, enhancing overall mental and emotional well-being.

Self-care practices are integral to maintaining a positive mindset. Prioritizing physical, emotional, and mental well-being through activities such as exercise, adequate sleep, and relaxation techniques contributes to resilience and optimism. By investing in self-care, individuals with epilepsy can better manage stress, reduce anxiety, and foster a positive mindset that supports overall recovery.

Embracing a positive mindset is a dynamic and intentional process that significantly influences the journey of epilepsy recovery. It involves reframing challenges, practicing mindfulness, cultivating gratitude, setting realistic goals, seeking social support, viewing setbacks as opportunities, and prioritizing self-care. This mindset not only enhances emotional well-being but also empowers individuals to navigate the complexities of epilepsy with resilience, adaptability, and a sense of purpose. As individuals embrace a positive mindset, they not only transform their relationship with epilepsy but also pave the way for a more fulfilling and empowered life beyond the condition.

Pursuing Your Dreams and Aspirations

Embarking on the journey of epilepsy recovery doesn't merely involve managing symptoms and adhering to medical advice; it's about reclaiming your life and rediscovering the pursuit of dreams and aspirations. While epilepsy might introduce challenges, it shouldn't serve as a barrier to your ambitions. In fact, overcoming adversity can infuse a unique strength and resilience into the pursuit of your goals.

Embracing Possibility

The first step in pursuing your dreams is to embrace the possibility that they are still achievable. Epilepsy may have altered the landscape of your life, but it doesn't negate your capacity for success and fulfillment. Recognize that your dreams may need to be approached with adaptability, but that doesn't diminish their significance or the impact they can have on your life.

Setting Realistic Goals

Setting realistic and achievable goals is a crucial aspect of pursuing your dreams amid epilepsy recovery. Break down your larger aspirations into smaller, manageable steps. This not only makes them less overwhelming but also allows you to celebrate incremental victories, fostering a positive mindset throughout the journey.

Building a Support System

Surrounding yourself with a supportive network is vital. Share your dreams and aspirations with those close to you, whether it's family, friends, or members of a support group. Their encouragement and understanding can provide the emotional backing you need to stay motivated and focused on your goals. Moreover, they can offer practical assistance during challenging times.

Mindfulness and Resilience

In the pursuit of your dreams, cultivating mindfulness and resilience becomes a powerful tool. Mindfulness practices, such as meditation and deep breathing, can help manage stress and anxiety, common challenges for individuals with epilepsy. Resilience enables you to bounce back from setbacks, viewing them as opportunities for learning and growth rather than insurmountable obstacles.

Seizing Opportunities

Epilepsy recovery doesn't mean avoiding opportunities; it means navigating them with awareness. Be open to seizing opportunities that align with your dreams, and communicate your needs effectively. Educate those around you about your condition, allowing for a supportive environment that accommodates your health requirements while enabling you to pursue your passions.

Adaptive Strategies

Adaptability is key when pursuing dreams amidst epilepsy recovery. Consider alternative strategies or pathways to reach your goals. This might involve finding creative solutions to accommodate potential challenges or adjusting timelines as needed. The ability to adapt ensures that setbacks don't derail your progress but rather become integral parts of your evolving journey.

Inspiring Stories

Drawing inspiration from individuals who have overcome similar challenges can be a powerful motivator. Seek out and connect with people who have pursued their dreams despite epilepsy. Their stories serve as a testament to the resilience of the human spirit and can provide valuable insights and advice for navigating your own path.

Celebrating Progress

Amid the pursuit of dreams, take time to celebrate your progress. Recognize and appreciate the milestones, both big and small. This positive reinforcement not only boosts your morale but also reinforces the idea that epilepsy recovery doesn't limit your capacity to achieve meaningful goals.

Professional Guidance

In some cases, seeking professional guidance can be instrumental in navigating the intersection of epilepsy recovery and pursuing aspirations. Consult with healthcare providers, therapists, or career counselors who understand the unique challenges you may face. They can offer tailored advice and strategies to help you achieve your dreams while prioritizing your health.

Pursuing your dreams and aspirations amid epilepsy recovery is a testament to your resilience and determination. By embracing the possibilities, setting realistic goals, building a strong support system, practicing mindfulness, seizing opportunities, adapting strategies, drawing inspiration from others, celebrating progress, and seeking professional guidance when needed, you can navigate this journey with confidence. Remember, epilepsy is a part of your story, but it doesn't define your capabilities or limit the fulfillment of your dreams. Your journey is unique, and your aspirations are within reach—embrace the adventure with courage and conviction.

Inspiring Stories of Epilepsy Triumphs

Epilepsy, with its unpredictable seizures, often poses daunting challenges. However, amidst the trials, many individuals have emerged triumphant, showcasing resilience, courage, and an unwavering spirit. These inspiring stories of epilepsy triumphs serve as beacons of hope for those navigating similar paths.

One remarkable tale is that of Sarah Thompson, who, despite facing epilepsy since childhood, refused to let it define her. Sarah experienced seizures that disrupted her education and social life, but her determination led her to explore alternative therapies. Embracing a holistic approach, she incorporated mindfulness practices and adopted a ketogenic diet, significantly reducing the frequency of her seizures. Sarah not only regained control of her health but also became an advocate for epilepsy awareness, inspiring others to explore diverse paths to recovery.

Another extraordinary journey is that of Mark Rodriguez, a professional athlete who confronted epilepsy head-on. Mark's seizures initially shattered his dreams of a sports career, but he refused to surrender to the limitations imposed by his condition. Through rigorous medical management and an unwavering commitment to fitness, Mark not only resumed his athletic pursuits but also excelled, eventually competing at an international level. His story underscores the transformative power of resilience and dedication in overcoming epilepsy's obstacles.

The narrative of Lisa Chen illuminates the strength found in community support. Diagnosed with epilepsy in her teens, Lisa initially grappled with feelings of isolation. However, by connecting with local epilepsy support groups, she discovered a network of individuals sharing similar experiences.

This support system provided emotional understanding and practical advice, empowering Lisa to confront challenges with newfound strength. Today, Lisa actively contributes to the epilepsy community, emphasizing the importance of solidarity in the journey toward triumph.

In the realm of arts and creativity, the story of Michael Turner stands out. Diagnosed with epilepsy in his twenties, Michael faced skepticism about pursuing a career in graphic design. Undeterred, he harnessed his unique perspective, using his experiences with epilepsy as a source of inspiration. Michael's innovative artwork not only garnered acclaim but also served as a powerful medium for epilepsy awareness. His story illustrates how adversity can fuel creativity, turning challenges into opportunities for personal and societal growth.

The account of Emma Carter exemplifies the role of education in epilepsy triumphs. Emma, diagnosed during her university years, encountered academic setbacks due to seizures. Instead of succumbing to despair, she collaborated with her professors to develop a personalized learning plan. Emma's persistence not only enabled her to complete her degree but also inspired institutional changes to accommodate students with epilepsy. Her story underscores the transformative impact of education and advocacy in overcoming obstacles.

These stories collectively reveal a mosaic of resilience, determination, and community that characterizes epilepsy triumphs. While each journey is unique, common threads of courage and perseverance tie them together. These individuals didn't merely endure their condition; they embraced it as a catalyst for personal growth, advocacy, and societal change.

In concluding these narratives of triumph, it is essential to recognize the strength inherent in the human spirit and the capacity to turn adversity into opportunities for empowerment. These inspiring stories serve as testaments to the fact that, with the right support, mindset, and resources, individuals living with epilepsy can not only manage their condition but also flourish, defying the limitations imposed by seizures. Their triumphs become a source of inspiration for others, fostering a sense of hope and possibility in the face of epilepsy's challenges.

Conclusion

Celebrating Your Epilepsy Recovery Journey

Embarking on the road to epilepsy recovery is a courageous and transformative journey, marked by resilience, self-discovery, and triumph over adversity. As you reach the conclusion of this profound expedition, it is essential to pause and celebrate the milestones, both big and small, that have defined your path to healing.

Reflecting on Progress:
Take a moment to reflect on how far you've come since the initial diagnosis. Consider the challenges you've faced, the treatments you've undergone, and the strength you've discovered within yourself. Acknowledge the progress you've made, recognizing that every step forward, no matter how modest, is a victory worth celebrating.

Embracing Personal Growth:
Epilepsy recovery extends beyond the physical aspects of managing seizures. It encompasses

personal growth and resilience. Reflect on the emotional and mental strength you've developed throughout this journey. Embrace the newfound wisdom, patience, and empathy that often accompany overcoming such obstacles.

Acknowledging Support Systems:
Celebrate the network of support that has surrounded you. Whether it's the unwavering encouragement of family, the understanding of friends, or the expertise of healthcare professionals, express gratitude for those who have been instrumental in your recovery. Consider organizing a gathering to share your appreciation and let them know how their support made a difference.

Documenting Milestones:
Create a visual representation of your journey by documenting key milestones. This could be a scrapbook, a journal, or a digital timeline. Include photos, quotes, and personal reflections to capture the highs and lows, showcasing the resilience that defines your epilepsy recovery narrative. Having a tangible reminder of your journey can be empowering and motivating.

Celebrating Resilience Events:

Host a celebration event to mark specific milestones in your recovery journey. Whether it's reaching a certain period without a seizure, successfully transitioning to a new treatment plan, or achieving a personal goal, these events can serve as powerful reminders of your strength and determination. Invite friends, family, and members of your support network to share in the joy of your accomplishments.

Expressing Gratitude:

Consider writing letters or notes of gratitude to those who have played a significant role in your recovery. Expressing your thanks not only strengthens your connections but also allows you to reflect on the positive impact others have had on your life. Gratitude can be a powerful tool for fostering a positive mindset and reinforcing your commitment to continued well-being.

Focusing on Self-Care:

Amidst the celebration, don't forget the importance of ongoing self-care. Your journey may continue to involve regular medical check-ups, self-monitoring, and maintaining a healthy lifestyle. Celebrate your recovery by prioritizing self-care activities that bring you joy and contribute to your overall well-being.

Inspiring Others:
Your recovery journey can serve as a beacon of hope for others facing similar challenges. Consider sharing your story through blogs, social media, or local support groups. By offering your experiences and insights, you contribute to a community of understanding and inspiration, fostering a sense of unity among those navigating their own paths to recovery.

In celebrating your epilepsy recovery journey, you not only honor the progress you've made but also inspire others and foster a sense of community. Each step taken, each obstacle overcome, is a testament to your strength and resilience. As you celebrate, remember that this journey is ongoing, and your commitment to well-being is a continuous source of empowerment and inspiration.

Moving Forward with Confidence

Recovery from epilepsy is a journey that extends far beyond the realm of medical treatments and seizure management. It's a transformational odyssey that requires resilience, self-discovery, and an unwavering commitment to living life to the fullest. As you traverse the path toward a renewed sense of well-being, moving forward with confidence becomes a pivotal theme, empowering individuals to embrace their journey and shape a future defined by strength and optimism.

Confidence in the context of epilepsy recovery is not just about the absence of seizures; it's a holistic approach encompassing physical, emotional, and social well-being. This chapter delves into the various facets of building confidence and seizing control of one's life after an epilepsy diagnosis.

1. Embracing Personal Growth:
Moving forward with confidence begins with a willingness to grow personally. Epilepsy, with its challenges, can serve as a catalyst for self-discovery. Individuals often unearth strengths and resilience they never knew they possessed. Recognizing and

embracing personal growth fosters a sense of empowerment that becomes the cornerstone of confidence.

2. Shifting Perspectives:

Confidence is intricately linked to the way we perceive challenges. Shifting perspectives from seeing epilepsy as a limitation to viewing it as a part of one's unique journey can be transformative. Understanding that overcoming obstacles contributes to personal development helps reshape the narrative surrounding epilepsy, paving the way for increased confidence.

3. Setting and Achieving Goals:

Nothing instills confidence like setting achievable goals and witnessing their realization. Whether it's mastering a new skill, pursuing education, or embracing a fulfilling career, setting and achieving goals creates a positive feedback loop. Small victories accumulate, leading to increased self-assurance and a sense of control over one's destiny.

4. Cultivating a Positive Mindset:

Confidence thrives in the soil of positivity. Cultivating a positive mindset involves consciously choosing optimism even in the face of adversity. Practicing gratitude, focusing on strengths, and acknowledging progress, no matter how small, contribute to building a reservoir of positivity that sustains confidence through the ups and downs of the recovery journey.

5. Establishing a Support System:

Confidence is not a solo endeavor. Establishing a robust support system is pivotal for navigating the challenges of epilepsy recovery. Surrounding oneself with understanding family, empathetic friends, and knowledgeable healthcare professionals creates a safety net that bolsters confidence. Shared experiences and mutual encouragement foster a sense of belonging and resilience.

6. Integrating Wellness Practices:

Physical and mental well-being are fundamental to confidence. Integrating wellness practices, such as regular exercise, nutritious diet, and stress management techniques, enhances overall health and resilience. A body and mind in balance contribute significantly to the assurance needed to face the uncertainties associated with epilepsy.

7. Facing Fear and Stigma:
Confidence is often tested in the face of fear and societal stigma. Confronting these challenges head-on, educating others about epilepsy, and dispelling myths contribute to the empowerment of individuals living with the condition. By challenging fear and stigma, individuals pave the way for greater acceptance, understanding, and, ultimately, confidence.

8. Celebrating Progress:
Amidst the ongoing journey, taking moments to acknowledge and celebrate progress is crucial. Every step forward, every triumph over a challenge, deserves recognition. Celebrating progress serves as a reminder of one's resilience and capability, reinforcing the foundation of confidence.

In conclusion, moving forward with confidence after an epilepsy diagnosis is a multi-faceted process that involves personal growth, positive mindset cultivation, and the establishment of a strong support system. It's about embracing the journey, setting and achieving goals, and facing challenges with resilience. Confidence is not a destination but a continuous evolution—a reflection of the strength and determination cultivated throughout the epilepsy recovery journey. As you move forward, remember that confidence is not the absence of challenges but the belief in your ability to overcome them. Embrace the journey, celebrate your victories, and step into the future with confidence and resilience.

Printed in Great Britain
by Amazon

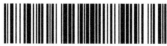

35883169R00066